THE
MEDITERRANEAN
DIET
for Beginners

CONTENTS

INTRODUCTION

When most people think about the word "diet," they think of deprivation and a lack of variety and excitement. With the Mediterranean diet, however, none of those characteristics apply.

The Mediterranean diet is filled with an almost unlimited assortment of fresh, delicious foods from all of the food groups. Although there is more of a focus on certain types of ingredients, none are excluded. People who eat a Mediterranean diet are able to enjoy the dishes they love, while also learning to appreciate how good the freshest, healthiest foods can be.

The Mediterranean diet is based primarily on the eating habits of people on the coasts of Italy, France, Morocco, Spain, and Greece. Because of their location and temperate climate, fresh vegetables, fruits, and seafood form the culinary foundation of these regions. You might think of eating the Mediterranean way as eating as though it's summer year-round. It also might remind you of meals you've enjoyed while at the beach or on an island vacation. Obviously, the Mediterranean diet is far from dull.

Following the Mediterranean diet, you'll not only enjoy fresh, delicious foods, you'll also take pleasure in knowing that you are feeding your body what is widely acknowledged as one of the healthiest diets on earth.

When eating well tastes like a yearlong vacation, it's easy and exciting to do.

$$\left(1\right)$$

UNDERSTANDING THE MEDITERRANEAN DIET

The Mediterranean diet has received a lot of media attention over the last few years, and for all the right reasons. The Mayo Clinic calls it the "heart-healthy diet," and it's considered to be among the most nutritious diets on the planet. Describing it as "a nutritional model that has remained constant over time and space," UNESCO recognized the Mediterranean diet as the Intangible Cultural Heritage of Spain, Italy, Greece, and Morocco in November 2010.

What Is the Mediterranean Diet?

Technically speaking, the Mediterranean diet is not a "diet" at all—it's a culinary tradition that focuses on fresh fruits and vegetables, whole grains, nuts, seafood, and olive oil, with the occasional glass of red wine. It's also part of a culture that appreciates and respects the freshest ingredients, simply prepared, and shares meals with friends and family in a leisurely and social way.

Everyone understands the importance of eating a well-balanced diet for better health and longevity, but very few people actually put it into practice. With most of our time being spent at work, we tend to look for quick and easy options when it comes to meals. These may include fast food, processed foods, and frozen dinners from the supermarket.

The Mediterranean diet is based on a simple premise: eat fresh, whole foods, in season. Over the years, many around the world have stopped eating seasonally because we can now get all kinds of produce year-round. What's more, making meals from scratch seems to require too much time out of our already overburdened schedules. As a result, our diets are full of processed foods, artificial ingredients, refined flour, unhealthful fats, and sugar.

The Mediterranean diet is simple and straightforward: eat less meat and more fish (especially those that have a high concentration of omega-3 fatty acids, which improve metabolism and help lower cholesterol and blood pressure), cook with olive oil, and eat fresh fruits and vegetables and whole grains several times a day. The Mediterranean diet also includes a daily serving of nuts, which have a high concentration of good-for-you monounsaturated and polyunsaturated fats.

Unlike many popular diets, eating the Mediterranean way does not require eliminating fat from your diet. It doesn't limit your fat consumption at all, in fact. With the Mediterranean diet, you simply replace all of the bad fats you eat with good fats such as olive oil, nuts, seeds, and avocados. Some studies suggest that a moderate intake of red wine can help lower the risk of heart disease, and the Mediterranean diet encourages wine consumption (up to five ounces per day for women under the age of sixty-five and ten ounces for men under the age of sixty-five).

To sum up the Mediterranean diet:

Eat lots of fruits and vegetables

Buy seasonal, fresh produce from your local farmers' market.

Go with whole grains

Replace foods made from white flour with whole-grain bread, cereal, and pasta. Include a variety of whole grains such as barley and millet, and choose brown rice over white.

Include a serving of nuts

Buy raw or roasted nuts such as almonds, cashews, and walnuts. (Walnuts are a rich source of omega-3 fatty acids.) Make nut butters at home or look for natural nut butters at your supermarket .

Replace the butter

Cook food in olive oil and use extra-virgin olive oil as a dip for breads and in salad dressings.

Use herbs and spices

Herbs and spices not only add a ton of flavor, allowing you to cut back on salt, but some also have antibacterial and anti-inflammatory properties.

Eat more fish

Salmon, sardines, anchovies, mackerel, and herring are some of the best sources of omega-3 fatty acids. Replace hamburgers and fried chicken with lightly sautéed or broiled fish.

Cut back on red meat

It's a well-known fact that red meat contributes to higher cholesterol and blood pressure. Replace steak with lean meats such as grilled fish and poultry.

Buy low-fat dairy products

Make sure that the cheese, milk, and yogurt you buy are low-fat. Choose 1 percent or 2 percent milk instead of whole milk, and low-fat frozen yogurt instead of ice cream.

The History of the Mediterranean Diet

The Mediterranean diet is not tied to a particular country. In fact, each region (Southern Italy, Spain, Greece, Southern France, and Morocco) has a different version of the diet, depending on the local produce and availability of ingredients. Sara Baer-Sinnott, president of the non-profit Oldways, points out that certain similarities do exist, such as the heavy consumption of fruits, vegetables, and olive oil. Preparation methods in these countries have remained the same for centuries—food is consumed fresh and is rarely deep-fried .

Dr. Ancel Keys first studied the Mediterranean diet when he was stationed in Salerno, Italy, in 1945. However, his work failed to garner attention until the fall of 1958, when Dr. Keys started his Seven Countries Study. This study examined the relationship between diet, lifestyle, stroke, and coronary heart disease in regions around the world. More than 12,000 men were enrolled in the study, which was conducted in seven countries in four regions (the United States, Southern Europe, Northern Europe, and Japan).

Data from the study indicated that deaths from coronary heart disease and stroke in the United States and Northern Europe greatly exceeded those in Southern Europe. Further research revealed a clear difference in the diet and lifestyle of these regions, information that eventually contributed to the popularity of the Mediterranean diet.

With the publication of several similar studies in the 1990s, the Mediterranean diet began to catch on in Western countries and has since become widely recognized as one of the healthiest in the world.

The Science behind the Mediterranean Diet

The model of most popular diet programs today is low fat, high protein. Not only is this model flawed, but it greatly limits the consumption of healthful fats, which the body needs to function properly. These healthful fats also serve to remove plaque buildup in arteries and keep the heart healthful by lowering the level of "bad" cholesterol.

Several studies have been conducted to determine exactly how healthful the Mediterranean diet is. While researchers have found the diet to be helpful in preventing a plethora of diseases, the most striking evidence points to its effectiveness in preventing heart disease.

Significant data is available via the Seven Countries Study, which found that people in Southern Europe suffered fewer deaths from coronary heart disease than people in the United States and Northern Europe.

A 2003 study conducted by the Harvard School of Public Health and the University of Athens Medical School in Athens, Greece, found that people who followed the Mediterranean diet had improved longevity over those who didn't.

Another study, conducted by the ***New England Journal of Medicine*** in 2008, found that people who followed the Mediterranean diet lost more weight than those who followed a low-carb or low-fat diet. And according to a recent study of 1.5 million healthy adults by the American Academy of Neurology, those who followed the Mediterranean diet were at a lower risk of heart disease and cognitive decline, such as Alzheimer's disease.

LIVING HEALTHIER AND LONGER ON THE MEDITERRANEAN DIET

The Mediterranean diet can help you lose unwanted weight, though it's far more than a weight-loss plan.

Numerous studies have documented the positive effects of the Mediterranean diet on coronary health and the risks of stroke, diabetes, and even some types of cancer. The health benefits of following the Mediterranean diet should be considered the most important reason to choose this nutritional lifestyle, and the impact of the diet doesn't stop with disease prevention. Because of its emphasis on avoiding processed foods and "bad" fats, the Mediterranean diet can help you shed unwanted pounds without calorie counting or strict rules.

Along with diet, the Mediterranean lifestyle involves regular, moderate exercise, which certainly helps with weight loss and also improves cardiovascular health and builds lean muscle. However, losing weight on the Mediterranean diet has nothing to do with a demanding physical regimen or lackluster meals devoid of your favorite foods. The diet is simple and straightforward and involves a vast array of delicious meals and snacks.

The more you learn about the Mediterranean diet, the more excited you will become about making this healthful lifestyle change.

The Incredible Health Benefits of Eating the Mediterranean Way

In February 2013, an article published in the **New England Journal of Medicine** made headlines in all of the country's major newspapers. The article, "Primary Prevention of Cardiovascular Disease with a Mediterranean Diet," detailed a five-year study on the health benefits of eating a Mediterranean diet, especially as it concerned coronary health and the risk of stroke.

In this latest clinical trial, over 7,000 people were divided into three groups. The first group of participants followed a Mediterranean diet and were also asked to consume at least one liter of extra-virgin olive oil per week. The second group also followed the Mediterranean diet, but they were asked to consume at least 30 grams of healthful nuts per week. The third group ate a low-fat Western diet. None of the participants was asked to exercise in any particular way and no calorie restrictions were placed on any of the groups.

At the end of the study, the results were newsworthy, indeed:

In this trial, an energy-unrestricted Mediterranean diet supplemented with either extra-virgin olive oil or nuts resulted in an absolute risk reduction of approximately 3 major cardiovascular events per 1000 person-years, for a relative risk reduction of approximately 30%, among high-risk persons who were initially free of cardiovascular disease. These results support the benefits of the Mediterranean diet for cardiovascular risk reduction. They are particularly relevant given the challenges of achieving and maintaining weight loss.

The study also reported that the risk of stroke was similarly reduced. In fact, it became so clear during the study that those on the Western diet were at an unhealthful disadvantage that the study was ended one year early due to moral and ethical concerns about asking that group to continue.

The results of this study were so dramatic and significant that they have garnered international attention. However, this is only one of many studies that demonstrate the health benefits of the Mediterranean diet. The scientific and medical communities have been praising it for years for its benefits to heart and artery health and kidney function; its reduction of the risk of stroke, type 2 diabetes, and metabolic syndrome; and even its prevention of some forms of cancer.

Research Supports the Many Health Benefits of the Mediterranean Diet

The Mediterranean diet's impact on heart health is one of its most commonly studied aspects, and there is copious research demonstrating its positive effect on coronary and vascular function .

In 2011, for example, researchers at the University of Miami published a study on the cardiovascular benefits of following a Mediterranean diet. The results of the study showed that consuming fresh fruit and vegetables, whole grains, olive oil, nuts, and fish was an excellent way to improve heart health and decrease the risk of cardiovascular disease.

Also in 2011, the journal **Public Health Nutrition** published the results of a study that demonstrated that the high volume of whole grains consumed in the Mediterranean diet makes it an effective method for reducing the risk of some forms of cancer, particularly colorectal cancer.

Then, in 2012, the Department of Internal Medicine and Geriatrics at the University of Palermo, Italy, published the results of a study that showed that the Mediterranean diet had a positive impact not only on heart health, but also on the incidence of diabetes.

And again in 2012, Spanish researchers from the Diabetes, Endocrinology, and Nutrition Unit of Dr. Josep Trueta Hospital in Girona reported that a study of 127 elderly men who ate either a Mediterranean diet with nuts, a Mediterranean diet with olive oil, or a low-fat diet revealed that after two years, both types of Mediterranean diet resulted in a significant improvement in bone health.

As you can see, the health benefits of the Mediterranean diet have been widely and comprehensively studied. Again and again, the Mediterranean diet is found to be an excellent way to improve heart, bone, and overall health and reduce the risk of cardiovascular disease, type 2 diabetes, metabolic syndrome, and some types of cancer.

The fact that it's a delicious way to eat that can also help you lose weight just makes the Mediterranean diet that much more appealing!

A Delicious Path to Weight Loss

One of the best ways to ensure that a diet will help you reach your weight-loss goals is to choose one that allows you to eat a wide variety of delicious foods and doesn't require you to go hungry, do without all of your favorite treats, or buy a lot of expensive and obscure ingredients. This is where the Mediterranean diet really stands out. There are no strict rules to follow and there is no deprivation or any need to drive all over town hunting down exotic ingredients or expensive supplements.

DID YOU KNOW? *Not only is the Mediterranean diet healthful and delicious, it can also be a very low-cost way to lose weight. The emphasis on eating whole foods (rather than processed) in season and shopping at farmers' markets means that you'll be buying produce at its peak of flavor and at the lowest prices. As everyone knows, an apple is cheaper than a strawberry in November, and it tastes better, too!*

How the Mediterranean Diet Can Help You Lose Weight

For many people who follow it, the Mediterranean diet results in weight loss in a natural and effortless way.

While most weight-loss diets focus on counting calories, following a strict menu, weighing and measuring foods, or undertaking a rigorous exercise program, the Mediterranean diet focuses on enjoying a wide variety of healthful foods and taking the time to savor meals and share them with others. It's a joyful way of eating as well as a healthful one.

By removing processed foods and fast foods from your diet, which are laden with unhealthful fats, sugar, and chemicals, you can significantly decrease your caloric intake while actually eating *more* food. Without counting calories or fat grams, you can trade unhealthful, "empty" foods for those that not only promote good health but also support the loss of stored fat.

For years, the low-fat diet has been promoted as the only real way to lose weight, but we now know that this just isn't true. In fact, a low-fat diet very often results in weight gain and can be unhealthful to boot.

A research hospital in Switzerland recently examined six separate studies comparing the Mediterranean diet and a low-fat diet. People who followed the Mediterranean diet for the studies experienced greater weight loss, lower body fat percentages, lower blood pressure, and better blood sugar levels than those on the low-fat diet.

Because it includes such a wide variety of healthful, fresh foods, the Mediterranean diet supplies a healthful amount of fiber and "good" fats, both of which support weight loss by helping you to feel full. A high-fiber diet also slows the rate at which sugar is absorbed into your bloodstream, which helps control both blood sugar and insulin levels. Too much insulin in the bloodstream stops fat loss, as insulin triggers fat storage. Fiber from whole grains, fruits, and vegetables also helps to improve digestion, which can be an important factor in weight loss. Many of the antioxidants found in fresh fruits and vegetables, such as lutein in apples, have also been shown to encourage weight loss.

Overall, the Mediterranean diet allows people to lose weight naturally and healthfully, without going hungry or eliminating food groups. You'll not only be able to lose weight on the diet, you'll enjoy yourself while you do.

(3)

STARTING THE MEDITERRANEAN DIET

Although the Mediterranean diet is straightforward, easy to follow, and delicious, your transition to the diet will be a lot easier and smoother if you do a little bit of preparation beforehand.

It's important that you have the right ingredients on hand, know about some of the foods you'll be eating, and have an idea of the meals you'd like to prepare. You'll also want to gradually (or immediately, if you're really eager) rid the house of the foods that you'll no longer be eating.

While there are no supplements or specially packaged foods to buy, there are several key ingredients that you'll need to stock up on, and you'll also want to locate sources for the freshest and most healthful fruits, vegetables, and fish.

Preparing for the Mediterranean diet is largely about preparing yourself for a new way of eating, adjusting your attitude toward food into one of joyful expectation and appreciation of good meals and good company. It's as much a mind-set as anything else, so you'll want to make your environment one in which the Mediterranean way of eating can be naturally followed and easily enjoyed.

Preparing for the Mediterranean diet can be as simple as getting out the good dishes so that you can fully enjoy your meals or visiting a few local markets to check out the freshness and prices of their offerings.

You can take a month to prepare your pantry and yourself, or you can take just a few days, but a little time spent in advance can make all the difference in those first few weeks of your healthful new lifestyle .

Planning Your Mediterranean Diet

With the Mediterranean diet, you don't need to run out and buy special appliances, hard-tofind or expensive ingredients, special supplements, or even new workout gear, but there are a few things that will make your transition to the diet easier and more fun.

Ease Your Way into More Healthful Eating

Before actually starting the diet, it can be helpful to spend a week or two cutting back on the least healthful foods that you currently eat. You might start with fast food if you frequent the drive-through, or eliminate cream-based sauces and soups. You can then start cutting back on processed foods like chips, boxed dinners, and frozen meals.

Some other things to start trimming might be sodas, coffee with a lot of milk and sugar, butter, and red meats such as beef, pork, and lamb. You don't have to eliminate these things entirely during this period, but you'd be surprised at how quickly your body adjusts if you gradually wean yourself from them. This can make it much easier to adapt to the diet once you do begin in earnest.

Start Thinking about What You'll Be Eating

When you're planning a vacation, you spend a lot of time looking through brochures, scanning websites, and reading books about your destination. It builds anticipation, informs you, and helps you make the best choices once you arrive. It's all part of the fun of traveling somewhere wonderful and new.

You should do the same thing while preparing to transition to the Mediterranean diet. Go through the information in Chapter 4 , including the shopping guide, and decide which foods you're most likely to eat so that you can collect appropriate recipes and meal ideas. Then read the recipes in Chapters 5 –9 and research some of the thousands of other Mediterranean meals that you can look forward to enjoying.

Gather What You'll Need

Everything in the Mediterranean diet is easily found at grocery stores, farmers' markets, and seafood shops .

Find out where your local farmers' markets are and spend a leisurely morning checking out what's available. Whenever possible, you'll want to buy seasonal fruits and vegetables, so talk to farmers about what they harvest and when. Small farmers love to talk about what they do and why they're so passionate about the food they grow. Building relationships with those vendors can lead not only to great new friendships, but also to getting special deals and the best selection, finding out ahead of time what's coming to market, and often some great recipes, too.

DID YOU KNOW? *Even urban areas are likely to have a CSA (Community Supported Agriculture) farm nearby. CSA farms are small, often family-owned farms that sell subscription packages of whatever they're growing that season. Many of these farms are organic and quite a few specialize in heirloom varieties of fruits and vegetables. For a moderate seasonal or weekly fee, the farm will supply you with enough of that week's harvest to feed your whole family. The contents of your share change with the seasons and include a variety of different items each week. Joining a CSA is a great way to enjoy the freshness and peak flavor that is so important to the Mediterranean diet, which is based on the diet of people who often get their veggies right out of their own gardens!*

The same is true of your local seafood market and butcher shop. Find out who is selling the freshest, most healthful meats and seafood and start building a relationship with those vendors.

When you're ready to start the diet, create a shopping list and get as many of your ingredients from your new sources as you can. If time is short or you're limited to the grocery store, the shopping guide in Chapter 4 can still help you make the best choices. Either way, you will want to have your refrigerator and cupboards stocked and ready to go before you begin. What you **don't** want is to resort to the drive-through or a takeout pizza because you didn't make it to the store.

In the next section, we'll share some great tips for making your Mediterranean diet a success, but if you take the above advice to heart, you'll be one step ahead.

The Top Ten Tips for Success

Here are the best ways, some large and some small, to help ensure that you enjoy your Mediterranean diet to the fullest. These strategies can also help you lose weight, if that's one of your goals, by making it easier for you to adjust to the diet and stick with it.

1. Treat Yourself Like Company

The Mediterranean diet is as much about **how** you eat as it is about **what** you eat. The Mediterranean people have a respect for and appreciation of food that inspires them to set beautiful (though often very simple) tables. Bring out the good china, put some fresh flowers in a canning jar, light some candles, or eat outside on the patio. However you choose to do it, treat every meal as though you were having guests.

2. Learn to Savor

In our fast-paced multitasking culture, we have a tendency to eat without paying attention to our food. We eat standing up or while driving to work, watching TV, or finishing up some paperwork. This is the antithesis of Mediterranean custom, where it's not uncommon to linger over even a simple meal for a couple of hours and where the idea of doing anything mundane while eating just seems silly.

Turn off the TV, even if you're eating alone. Put away the work, the cell phone, and any other distractions. Even if you're having dinner for one, focus on the delicious food you're eating. Really taste what's on your plate and start appreciating the pleasure of flavor.

3. Become a Social Eater

Gathering around food is something that families and friends do every day in the Mediterranean, even if all that's being served is some crusty bread with good olive oil. While Sunday afternoon dinners are traditionally an important part of the week in the Mediterranean region, even simple meals are an excuse to invite someone over for good food and conversation. Even when there are no guests, families will linger at the table to talk about the day and enjoy each other's presence.

Inviting friends and family over for a simple summer lunch or a casual dinner party is a great way to incorporate the Mediterranean approach to dining into your own life. For the Mediterranean people, eating is as much about the company as it is about the food, and meals really do taste better when you share them.

4. Learn to Make Substitutions

Very few things are off-limits in the Mediterranean diet, but moderation is key. If you're craving something you don't think you should be eating, like greasy French fries or salty potato chips, learn to make substitutions. You may find that the thing that stands in for your favorite junk food becomes your new favorite!

Kale chips taste better than commercial potato chips and they can be made without all of the unhealthful fat, excess salt, and preservatives. A refreshing homemade granita takes no time to make, the flavor is unparalleled, and it's much better for you than that ice cream you're used to.

5. Get Some Moderate Exercise Every Day—Preferably Outdoors

In the Mediterranean region, spending time outdoors is just a natural part of any day. Sunshine and good weather abound in the area, as do beautiful scenery and warm oceans. People spend as much time outside as they do inside, whether they're working in the garden, walking on the beach, or throwing a ball for the dog.

Try to get at least thirty minutes of moderate exercise three times per week. This has been shown to be an important element of losing weight, improving cardiovascular health, and attaining an overall feeling of happiness and well-being.

Try walking in the morning or after work, taking a ballroom dancing class, swimming in the pool or ocean, playing a game of catch with the kids, or any other activity that gets you moving. It doesn't have to be strenuous and it doesn't have to be the same activity every day—in fact, it shouldn't be.

6. Don't Tempt Yourself

Don't keep pastries in the pantry for visiting neighbors or chicken nuggets in the freezer just because they haven't expired yet. Having foods at home that are not part of the diet or that you tend to overindulge in is just tempting fate. If you need something to serve guests, the Mediterranean menu offers plenty of choices. There is no occasion for which you will need chicken nuggets. Give them to the family next door!

7. Don't Overwhelm Yourself

Try not to complicate your life by preparing three weeks' worth of menus at the get-go or trying ten new recipes in a week. Take things slowly, and cultivate a relaxed approach to your new way of eating. Try a few new recipes, but make sure they're not all complicated dishes that'll just stress you out. Most Mediterranean dishes are simple, with few ingredients and very straightforward preparation. You don't need a lot of fancy steps to make great meals.

8. Give Yourself a Break

So you snuck out to the fast-food place and ate the messiest and most calorie-laden burger they sell. Hopefully it was truly yummy. Now move on.

One slipup won't kill you. Do not spend three days eating garbage because you're upset about that slipup!

9. Try Something New Each Week

Eating the Mediterranean way should be fun, exciting, and even a little exotic. Try to choose one unfamiliar fruit, vegetable, fish, or other ingredient each week. It'll keep things interesting and enhance that sense of voyaging to another land.

10. Try Growing Your Own

The people of the Mediterranean region are very garden-focused. It's common for them to have lush kitchen gardens in their backyards, and even many city dwellers insist on a few pots of fresh herbs on the windowsill. Growing your own herbs and vegetables is fun, saves money, and is the best way to taste something at its very freshest.

(4)

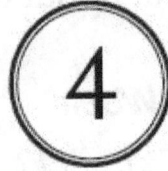

EATING ON THE MEDITERRANEAN DIET

At the heart of any successful diet are the foods that you will enjoy. Regardless of the rules or origin of a diet, it's important to know what you'll be eating and how best to prepare and enjoy your meals.

Happily, the Mediterranean diet offers wonderful variety and has very few "forbidden" items. Aside from replacing butter with olive oil, processed foods with fresh, and most meat with fish and plant-based proteins, there is very little that you have to sacrifice in order to follow the diet.

You can snack at will, enjoy delicious desserts, and visit your favorite restaurants on the Mediterranean diet, without counting calories or weighing your food.

Transitioning from a typical Western diet to the Mediterranean diet is all about learning how to shop for the freshest ingredients and reorganizing your daily food pyramid to emphasize fresh fruits and vegetables, healthful fats, and seafood over meat and starch.

It's an easy transition to make, and most people find that within a few weeks they are looking forward to their meals and learning to savor them in a way that they hadn't before.

What's on Your Plate?

The traditional Western diet is very low in fresh fruits and vegetables and very high in starchy foods and red meat. In contrast, the Mediterranean diet is based largely on fresh produce, with whole grains at most meals, seafood several times per week, and meat only a few times per month, usually in small portions .

Olive oil is used far more often than butter, and cream-based sauces, salad dressings, and soups are very rarely eaten. Instead, meals may include tomato-based sauces, vinaigrettes, and clear soups.

While no meat is forbidden on the Mediterranean diet, it is not the staple that it is in the Western world. It's more often served as a side dish or used as flavoring than it is an entrée by itself. Poultry is eaten more than beef, pork, or lamb, and eggs are a more common source of protein than is meat.

Here is what your typical daily diet should look like:

Fresh fruits and vegetables: *Unlimited, but at least 4 servings per day*

All fruits and vegetables are allowed on the Mediterranean diet and in unlimited quantities. The only exceptions are corn and white potatoes, which should be eaten in very limited amounts, as they are very starchy.

Eating your fruits and vegetables raw is great, but steamed, roasted, sautéed, poached, grilled, and baked fruits and vegetables are all welcome on the Mediterranean diet. Avoid boiling vegetables, as many of the nutrients are lost in the water and the result is far less flavorful and colorful than with other cooking methods. Use olive oil and herbs in the preparation rather than butter and excessive salt.

Whole grains: *3 to 5 servings per day*

Whole grains are an integral part of the Mediterranean diet and part of the reason that the diet is so rich in heart-healthful fiber. Forgo white bread and overly processed grain products and focus on whole grains such as whole wheat, oats, barley, and brown rice. Whole-grain pasta is perfectly fine, but portion sizes are much smaller in the Mediterranean than they are in the United States. Heaping plates of pasta aren't common in Italy; rather, pasta is used as a backdrop for a flavorful sauce and plenty of vegetables.

Healthful fats: *4 to 6 servings per day*

Healthful fats are an essential part of the Mediterranean diet. Get them from olive oil, olives, avocados, fresh fish and shellfish, nuts, and seeds.

DID YOU KNOW? *Not all olive oils are created equal. Extra-virgin olive oil is cold-processed and comes from the first pressing of the olives, so it is the most expensive. Virgin olive oil is from subsequent pressings, so it usually lacks the pure flavor of extra-virgin, but it's unrefined, which is good. Olive oil is a combination of virgin olive oil and refined olive oil. It's cheaper and has a stronger flavor, but it contains fewer omega-3 fats. Opt for virgin and extra-virgin instead. If price is a concern, use extra-virgin only for fresh eating on salads and vegetables and virgin for cooking. Light olive oil refers to the flavor, not the fat, and should be used for baking cakes and cookies, where the flavor of a stronger olive oil might be unwelcome.*

Fish and seafood: *At least 3 servings per week*

Cold-water, fatty fishes such as salmon, sardines, cod, haddock, and mackerel are highest in omega-3 fats. You may also enjoy shellfish such as mussels, clams, oysters, shrimp, crab, and lobster.

Dairy products: *Up to 7 servings per week*

Milk, yogurt, and cheese are welcome on the Mediterranean diet, but they are not eaten in the high quantities common in the Western diet. Choose low-fat cheeses and milk and opt for Greek yogurt whenever possible, as it contains twice the protein of regular yogurt. Generally, milk is reserved for cereal, coffee or tea, and baking. Cheese is used as a dessert or as a flavoring for soups, salads, and entrées, and cheese sauces are not a regular part of the Mediterranean diet.

Red wine: *Up to one 5-ounce glass per day for women, two glasses per day for men*

Red wine is an important part of the Mediterranean diet and is typically enjoyed with the afternoon or evening meal, rather than on its own. The antioxidants in red wine, particularly resveratrol, are credited with improved heart health and slowed cellular aging. If you don't care for wine, try to get in several servings of red or purple fruits per week, such as grapes, raspberries, blackberries, and plums.

Eggs: *3 to 5 servings (of two eggs each) per week*

Eggs are traditionally enjoyed frequently in the Mediterranean diet, especially by those families that raise their own chickens. Opt for organic, free-range, hormone-free eggs. They're safer and contain more omega-3 fats than commercial eggs. Use them for baking, in sauces, and as entrées.

Poultry: *2 to 5 servings per week*

Poultry is eaten far more often in the Mediterranean than red meat. You can eat any cuts of chicken and turkey, although it's recommended that you remove the skin and any visible fat before eating. Game birds are also welcome on the diet, so you can choose quail, duck, pheasant, pigeon, or any other bird that you like.

Sweets: *Up to 4 servings per week*

Although the people of the Mediterranean enjoy sweets, dessert is typically cheese and/or fruit, not sugary pastries. Go for fruit most of the week and reserve sweeter desserts for special meals with guests or as an occasional treat. Artificial sweeteners are not recommended; instead, stick with sugar, honey, and molasses in small quantities.

Red meat: *3 to 5 servings per month*

Red meats such as beef, pork, and lamb are generally reserved for a few special meals, and portions are much smaller than on most Western plates. Choose organic, grass-fed meats whenever possible (as they are higher in omega-3s), and leaner cuts such as sirloin or loin should be given preference over the fattier ones, such as bacon or ribs. A 3to 5-ounce steak is plenty for one meal, as opposed to a gigantic rib eye. You can also stretch your portions by using red meat as part of a hearty stew or as an ingredient in salads and soups.

A word about salt

As part of a heart-healthful meal plan, the Mediterranean diet is fairly low in sodium. Limit the use of table salt and rely on fresh herbs and a variety of spices to flavor your food .

As you can see, there's plenty to eat in the Mediterranean diet, and few things are offlimits or even dramatically limited. You'll be able to satisfy your appetite while improving your health and even losing weight.

Your Mediterranean Shopping Guide

While you can do all of your shopping at your favorite supermarket, getting at least some fresh items from your local farmers' market, seafood shop, and butcher is an enjoyable way to source your food as well as a better bet for getting the freshest ingredients.

When you do shop at the grocery store, try to stay in the perimeter of the store as much as possible. This means getting the vast majority of your food from the produce, seafood, bulk foods, meat, and dairy aisles.

The center aisles of the grocery store are generally filled with processed foods and unhealthful snacks, although you'll need to venture into them to purchase some of your grains, condiments, oils, pasta, spices, and other staples. Keep your shopping list in hand so you don't stray!

The **produce section** or the farmers' market is where you really want to fill your cart. Choose organic fruits and vegetables as much as possible and get a wide variety of colors into your cart each week to keep things interesting and maximize your antioxidant intake. Opt for in-season produce more often than out-of-season, as those items have been picked too soon and shipped too far to be at peak flavor.

In the **seafood section** or at the seafood shop, get to know the fishmonger. He or she will be able to tell you what is freshest, help you choose the most heart-healthful varieties, and even give you cooking tips. Look for cold-water fish such as salmon, mackerel, cod, haddock, and sardines and fresh shellfish such as mussels, clams, oysters, shrimp, crab, and lobster. Frozen fish is fine if it's more affordable or more readily available, but skip the breaded or fried versions.

At the **meat counter** , choose skinless poultry and lean cuts of red meat such as those from the loin. Organic, grass-fed meats are preferred as they're free of harmful chemicals and hormones and higher in omega-3 fats. Have the butcher trim any visible fat for you.

In the **dairy aisle** , choose low-fat or fat-free versions of cheese, yogurt, and milk. (You'll be getting plenty of healthful fats from olive oil, nuts, and seeds.) Try to do without butter as much as is possible, but butter is preferable over margarine, which contains hydrogenated oils and trans fats .

In the **freezer section** , you can supplement your fresh produce and seafood supplies if there is something you'd like that is currently out of season. While fresh is best, frozen peaches picked at the peak of ripeness are far better than canned peaches or those picked green and shipped for thousands of miles. Again, when buying seafood, skip the fried, battered, or buttered preparations. The same goes for chicken.

In the **center of the store** , you'll want to focus on staples and leave the majority of the shelves alone. Whole-grain flour, oats, unsalted and unsweetened nuts and seeds (especially walnuts, almonds, cashews, and pumpkin seeds), olive oil and olives, rice, pasta, spices, and whole-grain cereals and pastas are some of the products you'll want to stock up on.

You may need a few weeks to get used to shopping the Mediterranean way, but once you do, you'll find that circling the store and avoiding the processed-food aisles will actually cut down on the time it takes to purchase your weekly groceries—and will probably lower your bill as well.

Eating Out on the Mediterranean Diet

Eating out on the Mediterranean diet is very easy, and the trend toward healthier menus and vegetarian and vegan offerings makes it easier than ever before.

Some of the best restaurants for the Mediterranean diet are seafood houses, farm-to-table establishments, and Italian, Spanish, Greek, and Provençal (Southern French) restaurants. Vegetarian restaurants also offer a wide variety of delicious pasta dishes and entrées that are made healthfully and with fresh ingredients.

Here are a few guidelines to follow when dining out on the Mediterranean diet:

- Go easy on the bread basket. Although bread is welcomed on the Mediterranean diet, you don't want to add too many calories to your meal before your entrée hits the table. When you do eat bread, ask that olive oil and pepper be brought to the table instead of butter.
- Order food that is broiled, baked, sautéed (in olive oil, not butter), grilled, braised, roasted, poached, or steamed. Avoid any entrée that is breaded or deep-fried.
- Try to include a fresh salad with your meal, but skip the creamy dressings. Instead, ask for vinaigrette or olive oil and vinegar.
- If you order a meat entrée, chances are that the portion will be much larger than those favored on the Mediterranean diet. This is also usually true when having pasta. If this is the case, ask the server to either box half of it up before serving you or to bring you a carryout box along with the entrée. Then just put about half of the portion into the

box before you start eating and enjoy it another day. This will stretch your dollar without stretching your waistline.

- For the most part, opt for fruit or a cheese plate for dessert. Other good choices for a sweet treat are sorbet and baked fruit dishes. By all means, have a piece of chocolate cake or a crème brûlée now and then, but make it a rare treat and share it with someone or take half of it home.

The Mediterranean diet is all about enjoying great food in pleasant surroundings and with wonderful people. This makes restaurant dining a natural part of the diet, so try not to stress too much about where and what to eat. Most restaurants have plenty of Mediterraneanfriendly choices.

Seven-Day Sample Meal Plan

What follows is a sample of a week's worth of menus to give you an idea of how well you can eat on the Mediterranean diet and to help you start thinking about your meal plan. You need to get at least the minimum recommended servings from each food group. Choose water for most of your beverages, although coffee and tea are fine in moderation. If you drink wine, try to have a glass of red wine with your dinner or weekend lunch at least a few times per week.

Items marked with an asterisk (*) are included in the recipes section.

Monday

Breakfast
Berry Breakfast Smoothie *

Lunch
Garden salad with vinaigrette

Whole-grain roll or toast

Snack
Fresh apple

Mozzarella cheese stick

Dinner
Dilly Baked Salmon *

Sautéed spinach

Baked sweet potato with olive oil and pepper

Dessert
Summer Fruit Granita *

Tuesday

Breakfast
Whole-grain cereal with low-fat milk
Fresh peach or nectarine

Lunch
Greek Chicken Salad *
Whole-grain roll or toast
Fresh watermelon

Snack
Nutty Apple Salad *

Dinner
Fettuccine with Tomatoes and Pesto
* Spinach salad with vinaigrette

Dessert
Home-Baked Biscotti *

Wednesday

Breakfast

Mediterranean Omelet *
Whole-grain English muffin or toast

Lunch

Savory Avocado Spread *
Whole-grain crackers
Cup of minestrone soup

Snack

Kale Chips *

Dinner

Grilled chicken breast
Roasted root vegetables
Garden salad
Whole-grain roll

Dessert

Fresh fruit and cheese

Thursday

Breakfast
Hearty Berry Breakfast Oats *

Lunch
Fresh Tomato Pasta Bowl *
Sliced fresh cantaloupe

Snack
Café Cooler *

Dinner
Flank Steak Spinach Salad *
Whole-grain roll

Dessert
Grilled Pineapple and Melon *

Friday

Breakfast
Summer Day Fruit Salad *
Soft-boiled eggs
Whole-grain toast

Lunch
Roasted Vegetable Soup *
Whole-grain crackers
Fresh peach

Snack
Spicy-Sweet Roasted Walnuts *
Fresh apple

Dinner
Mussels with White Wine *
Sautéed green beans and mushrooms
Crusty whole-grain baguette

Dessert
Baked Pears in Red Wine Sauce *

Saturday

Breakfast
Egg, Pancetta, and Spinach Benedict *
Cup of fresh strawberries and blueberries

Lunch
Fruited Chicken Salad *
Whole-grain English muffin or roll

Snack
Greek yogurt

Dinner
Oven-Poached Cod *
Broiled tomatoes with Parmesan cheese
Sautéed kale
Whole-grain dinner roll or baguette

Dessert
Chocolate-Dipped Fruit Bites *

Sunday

Breakfast
Scrambled eggs
Fresh pineapple
Whole-grain toast

Lunch
Garlicky Broiled Sardines *
Crusty whole-grain baguette
Garden salad with vinaigrette

Snack
Citrus-Kissed Melon *
Unsalted walnuts

Dinner
Herb-Roasted Whole Chicken *
Grilled endive
Garlic risotto
Spinach salad with vinaigrette

Dessert
Red Grapefruit Granita *

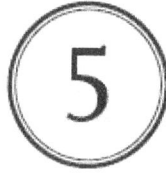

Berry Breakfast Smoothie

What a great way to enjoy a healthful and filling breakfast even on your busiest mornings! The Greek yogurt supplies a meal's worth of low-fat protein that will keep you going all morning.

- 1/2 cup vanilla low-fat Greek yogurt
- 1/4 cup low-fat milk

- 1/2 cup fresh or frozen blueberries or strawberries (or a combination)
- 6 to 8 ice cubes

Place the Greek yogurt, milk, and berries in a blender and blend until the berries are liquefied. Add the ice cubes and blend on high until thick and smooth. Serve immediately.

Serves 1.

Mediterranean Omelet

If you chop your vegetables the night before, this omelet comes together very quickly. Feel free to use any vegetables that happen to be in season or need to be used up.

- 2 teaspoons extra-virgin olive oil, divided
- 1 garlic clove, minced
- 1/2 red bell pepper, thinly sliced
- 1/2 yellow bell pepper, thinly sliced
- 1/4 cup thinly sliced red onion
- 2 tablespoons chopped fresh basil
- 2 tablespoons chopped fresh parsley, plus extra for garnish
- 1/2 teaspoon salt
- 1/2 teaspoon freshly ground black pepper
- 4 large eggs, beaten

In a large, heavy skillet, heat 1 teaspoon of the olive oil over medium heat. Add the garlic, peppers, and onion to the pan and sauté, stirring frequently, for 5 minutes.

Add the basil, parsley, salt, and pepper, increase the heat to medium-high, and sauté for 2 minutes. Slide the vegetable mixture onto a plate and return the pan to the heat.

Heat the remaining 1 teaspoon olive oil in the same pan and pour in the beaten eggs, tilting the pan to coat evenly. Cook the eggs just until the edges are bubbly and all but the center is dry, 3 to 5 minutes.

Either flip the omelet or use a spatula to turn it over.

Spoon the vegetable mixture onto one-half of the omelet and use a spatula to fold the empty side over the top. Slide the omelet onto a platter or cutting board.

To serve, cut the omelet in half and garnish with fresh parsley.

Serves 2.

Hearty Berry Breakfast Oats

Whole-grain oats and fresh berries provide a hefty dose of fiber, and the combination is not only nutritious but delicious as well. The fresh berries also supply vitamin C and other antioxidants, and the walnuts provide a serving of omega-3 fats.

- 11/2 cups whole-grain rolled or quickcooking oats (not instant)
- 3/4 cup fresh blueberries, raspberries, or blackberries, or a combination
- 2 teaspoons honey
- 2 tablespoons walnut pieces

Prepare the whole-grain oats according to the package directions and divide between 2 deep bowls.

In a small microwave-safe bowl, heat the berries and honey for 30 seconds. Top each bowl of oatmeal with the fruit mixture. Sprinkle the walnuts over the fruit and serve hot.

Serves 2.

Garden Scramble

Similar to a frittata, this savory breakfast dish is a great way to use up small amounts of fresh vegetables. You can also make this with any leftover grilled vegetables you may have lingering from a recent dinner.

- 1 teaspoon extra-virgin olive oil
- 1/2 cup diced yellow squash
- 1/2 cup diced green bell pepper
- 1/4 cup diced sweet white onion
- 6 cherry tomatoes, halved
- 1 tablespoon chopped fresh basil
- 1 tablespoon chopped fresh parsley
- 1/2 teaspoon salt
- 1/4 teaspoon freshly ground black pepper
- 8 large eggs, beaten

In a large nonstick skillet, heat the olive oil over medium heat. Add the squash, pepper, and onion and sauté until the onion is translucent, 3 to 4 minutes.

Add the tomatoes, basil, and parsley and season with salt and pepper. Sauté for 1 minute, then pour the beaten eggs over the vegetables. Cover the pan and reduce the heat to low.

Cook until the eggs are cooked through, 5 to 6 minutes, making sure that the center is no longer runny.

To serve, slide the frittata onto a platter and cut into wedges.

Serves 4.

Summer Day Fruit Salad

Nothing says "summer" quite like a big, colorful fruit salad. This one combines coconut, melon, and berries for a delicious medley of flavors. It will keep for up to three days if stored in a covered container in the refrigerator, so it's a great dish to make in advance for work lunches and weekday snacking.

- 2 cups cubed honeydew melon
- 2 cups cubed cantaloupe
- 2 cups red seedless grapes
- 1 cup sliced fresh strawberries
- 1 cup fresh blueberries
- Zest and juice of 1 large lime

- 1/2 cup unsweetened toasted coconut flakes
- 1/4 cup honey
- 1/4 teaspoon salt
- 1/2 cup extra-virgin olive oil

Combine all of the fruits, the lime zest, and the coconut flakes in a large bowl and stir well to blend. Set aside.

In a blender, combine the lime juice, honey, and salt and blend on low. Once the honey is incorporated, slowly add the olive oil and blend until opaque.

Pour the dressing over the fruit and mix well. Cover and refrigerate for at least 4 hours before serving, stirring a few times to distribute the dressing.

Serves 8.

Egg, Pancetta, and Spinach Benedict

This is a breakfast dish for weekend mornings, when you have more time to linger over your meal. Although pancetta (Italian-style unsmoked bacon) should be reserved as an occasional treat, a little bit of it delivers a large helping of flavor. If you can't find pancetta, you can substitute unsmoked bacon, which is sold near the salt pork in most stores.

- 1/4 cup diced pancetta
- 2 cups baby spinach leaves
- 1/4 teaspoon freshly ground black pepper
- 1/4 teaspoon salt, or to taste
- 2 large eggs
- Extra-virgin olive oil (optional)
- 1 whole-grain English muffin, toasted

In a medium, heavy skillet, brown the pancetta over medium-low heat for about 5 minutes, stirring frequently, until crisp on all sides.

Stir in the spinach, pepper, and salt if desired (it may not need any, depending on how salty the pancetta is). Cook, stirring occasionally, until the spinach is just wilted, about 5 minutes. Transfer the mixture to a medium bowl.

Crack the eggs into the same pan (add olive oil if the pan looks dry), and cook until the whites are just opaque, 3 to 4 minutes. Carefully flip the eggs and continue cooking for 30 seconds to 1 minute until done to your preferred degree for over-easy eggs.

Place a muffin half on each of 2 plates and top each with half of the spinach mixture and 1 egg, yolk side up. Pierce the yolks just before serving.

Serves 2.

Peach Sunrise Smoothie

Here's a quick breakfast idea for those mornings when a sit-down meal is out of the question. The Greek yogurt supplies a healthful amount of protein to satisfy you until lunch. If peaches are out of season, frozen peaches will do nicely.

- 1 large unpeeled peach, pitted and sliced (about 1/2 cup)
- 6 ounces vanilla or peach low-fat Greek yogurt
- 2 tablespoons low-fat milk
- 6 to 8 ice cubes

Combine all ingredients in a blender and blend until thick and creamy. Serve immediately.

Serves 1.

Oat and Fruit Parfait

A parfait is a great way to get a serving of whole grains into your breakfast without relying on toast or cereal. The toasted oat and nut mixture will keep for several weeks in an airtight container, so feel free to make a large batch to have on hand for meals and snacks.

- 1/2 cup whole-grain rolled or quickcooking oats (not instant)
- 1/2 cup walnut pieces
- 1 teaspoon honey

- 1 cup sliced fresh strawberries
- 11/2 cups (12 ounces) vanilla low-fat Greek yogurt
- Fresh mint leaves for garnish

Preheat the oven to 300°F.

Spread the oats and walnuts in a single layer on a baking sheet.

Toast the oats and nuts just until you begin to smell the nuts, 10 to 12 minutes. Remove the pan from the oven and set aside.

In a small microwave-safe bowl, heat the honey just until warm, about 30 seconds. Add the strawberries and stir to coat.

Place 1 tablespoon of the strawberries in the bottom of each of 2 dessert dishes or 8-ounce glasses. Add a portion of yogurt and then a portion of oats and repeat the layers until the containers are full, ending with the berries. Serve immediately or chill until ready to eat.

Serves 2.

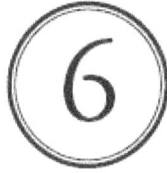

Greek Chicken Salad

The tartness of feta cheese is a nice counterpoint to mild chicken breast, salty olives, and sweet cherry tomatoes. The chicken mixture will keep well for up to three days in a covered container in the fridge, and the flavors intensify as it sits, so this is a good dish to make ahead.

- 1/4 cup balsamic vinegar
- 1 teaspoon freshly squeezed lemon juice
- 1/4 cup extra-virgin olive oil
- 1/4 teaspoon salt
- 1/4 teaspoon freshly ground black cheese pepper
- 2 grilled boneless, skinless chicken breasts, sliced (about 1 cup)
- 1/2 cup thinly sliced red onion
- 10 cherry tomatoes, halved
- 8 pitted Kalamata olives, halved
- 2 cups roughly chopped romaine lettuce
- 1/2 cup feta

In a medium bowl, combine the vinegar and lemon juice and stir well. Slowly whisk in the olive oil and continue whisking vigorously until well blended. Whisk in the salt and pepper.

Add the chicken, onion, tomatoes, and olives and stir well. Cover and refrigerate for at least 2 hours or overnight.

To serve, divide the romaine between 2 salad plates and top each with half of the chickenvegetable mixture. Top with feta cheese and serve immediately.

Serves 2.

Savory Avocado Spread

You'll find many lunchtime uses for this versatile spread. On toasted whole-grain bread, it makes a delicious sandwich. You can also add cooked seafood to create a mayo-less seafood salad, spread it on crackers, or use it as a dip for fresh vegetables. It will keep in an airtight container in the refrigerator for up to one day without browning.

- 1 ripe avocado, peeled and pitted
- 1 teaspoon freshly squeezed lemon juice
- 6 boneless sardine filets (packed in olive oil)
- 1/4 cup diced sweet white onion
- 1 stalk celery, diced
- 1/2 teaspoon salt
- 1/4 teaspoon freshly ground black pepper

In a blender or food processor, combine the avocado, lemon juice, and sardine filets and pulse just until fairly smooth. A few chunks are fine for texture.

Spoon the mixture into a small bowl and add the onion, celery, salt, and pepper. Mix well with a fork and serve as desired.

Makes 11/2 cups.

Cheesy Stuffed Tomatoes

This dish reheats well if you'd like to make it ahead to take to work. It's a nice change from a salad or sandwich and also makes a lovely summer brunch entrée.

- 4 large, ripe tomatoes
- 1 tablespoon extra-virgin olive oil
- 2 garlic cloves, minced
- 1/2 cup diced yellow onion
- 1/2 pound white or cremini mushrooms, sliced
- 1 tablespoon chopped fresh basil
- 1 tablespoon chopped fresh oregano
- 1/2 teaspoon salt
- 1/4 teaspoon freshly ground black pepper
- 1 cup shredded part-skim mozzarella cheese
- 1 tablespoon grated Parmesan cheese

Preheat the oven to 375°F. Line a baking sheet with aluminum foil.

Slice a sliver from the bottom of each tomato so they will stand upright without wobbling. Cut a 1/2-inch slice from the top of each tomato and use a spoon to gently remove most of the pulp, placing it in a medium bowl. Place the tomatoes on the baking sheet.

In a medium, heavy skillet, heat the olive oil over medium heat. Sauté the garlic, onion, mushrooms, basil, and oregano for 5 minutes, and season with salt and pepper.

Transfer the mixture to the bowl and blend well with the tomato pulp. Stir in the mozzarella cheese.

Fill each tomato loosely with the mixture, top with Parmesan cheese, and bake until the cheese is bubbly, 15 to 20 minutes. Serve immediately.

Serves 2.

Roasted Vegetable Soup

Cooler weather calls for this wonderfully rich, comforting, and flavorful soup. It keeps well in the fridge for as long as a week and freezes well in individual containers, ready to defrost for a quick meal anytime.

- 2 sweet potatoes, peeled and sliced
- 2 parsnips, peeled and sliced
- 2 carrots, peeled and sliced
- 2 tablespoons extra-virgin olive oil
- 1 teaspoon chopped fresh rosemary
- 1 teaspoon chopped fresh thyme
- 1 teaspoon salt
- 1/2 teaspoon freshly ground black pepper
- 4 cups vegetable or chicken broth
- Grated Parmesan cheese for garnish (optional)

Preheat the oven to 400°F. Line a baking sheet with aluminum foil.

In a large bowl, combine the sweet potatoes, parsnips, and carrots. Add the olive oil and toss to coat. Add the rosemary, thyme, salt, and pepper, tossing well.

Spread out the vegetables on the baking sheet and roast until tender and brown at the edges, 30 to 35 minutes. Remove the baking sheet from the oven and allow to cool until just warm.

Working in batches, transfer some of the vegetables and broth to a blender or food processor and blend until smooth. Pour each blended batch into a large saucepan.

When all of the vegetables have been puréed, heat the soup over low heat just until heated through. To serve, ladle into bowls and top with Parmesan cheese if desired.

Serves 6.

Pesto-Glazed Chicken Breasts

A savory pesto topping elevates chicken to a new level of flavor that will quickly make this one of your favorite meals. You'll have leftover pesto, which can be used to top a pasta side dish for the chicken or stored in a covered container in the fridge for up to a week.

- 1/4 cup plus 1 tablespoon extra-virgin olive oil, divided
- 4 boneless, skinless chicken breasts
- 1/2 teaspoon salt
- 1/4 teaspoon freshly ground black pepper

- 1 packed cup fresh basil leaves
- 1 garlic clove, minced
- 1/4 cup grated Parmesan cheese
- 1/4 cup pine nuts

In a large, heavy skillet, heat 1 tablespoon of the olive oil over medium-high heat.

Season the chicken breasts on both sides with salt and pepper and place in the skillet. Cook for 10 minutes on the first side, then turn and cook for 5 minutes.

Meanwhile, in a blender or food processor, combine the basil, garlic, Parmesan cheese, and pine nuts, and blend on high. Gradually pour in the remaining 1/4 cup olive oil and blend until smooth.

Spread 1 tablespoon pesto on each chicken breast, cover the skillet, and cook for 5 minutes. Serve the chicken pesto side up.

Serves 4.

Fresh Tomato Pasta Bowl

Pasta entrées don't have to be smothered with heavy meat or cream sauces. In fact, along Italy's Mediterranean coast, lighter sauces are the norm. This is a perfect pasta dish for lunchtime, when a heavier meal would weigh you down.

- 8 ounces whole-grain linguine
- 1 tablespoon extra-virgin olive oil
- 2 garlic cloves, minced
- 1/4 cup chopped yellow onion
- 1 teaspoon chopped fresh oregano
- 1/2 teaspoon salt
- 1/4 teaspoon freshly ground black pepper
- 1 teaspoon tomato paste
- 8 ounces cherry tomatoes, halved
- 1/2 cup grated Parmesan cheese
- 1 tablespoon chopped fresh parsley

Bring a large saucepan of water to a boil over high heat and cook the linguine according to the package instructions until al dente (still slightly firm). Drain, reserving 1/2 cup of the pasta water. Do not rinse the pasta.

In a large, heavy skillet, heat the olive oil over medium-high heat. Sauté the garlic, onion, and oregano until the onion is just translucent, about 5 minutes.

Add the salt, pepper, tomato paste, and 1/4 cup of the reserved pasta water. Stir well and allow it to cook for 1 minute.

Stir in the tomatoes and cooked pasta, tossing everything well to coat. Add more pasta water if needed.

To serve, mound the pasta in shallow bowls and top with Parmesan cheese and parsley.

Serves 4.

Garlicky Broiled Sardines

Even if you're not in love with sardines straight from the can, you might find yourself loving this dish. It's deliciously garlicky and quite addictive. As a bonus, it's ready in about five minutes. If you buy sardines canned in olive oil, you can omit the olive oil in the recipe.

- 4 (3.25-ounce) cans sardines (about 16 sardines), packed in water or olive oil
- 2 tablespoons extra-virgin olive oil (if sardines are packed in water)
- 4 garlic cloves, minced
- 1/2 teaspoon red pepper flakes
- 1/2 teaspoon salt
- 1/4 teaspoon freshly ground black pepper

Preheat the broiler. Line a baking dish with aluminum foil. Arrange the sardines in a single layer on the foil.

Combine the olive oil (if using), garlic, and red pepper flakes in a small bowl and spoon over each sardine. Season with salt and pepper.

Broil just until sizzling, 2 to 3 minutes.

To serve, place 4 sardines on each plate and top with any remaining garlic mixture that has collected in the baking dish.

Serves 4.

Fruited Chicken Salad

A satisfying blend of savory and sweet, creamy and crunchy, this lunch dish is a quick way to use up leftover cooked chicken breast. Serve on bread or toast for a traditional sandwich, or spoon into an avocado half for a delicious salad.

- 2 cups chopped cooked chicken breast
- 2 Granny Smith apples, peeled, cored, and diced
- 1/2 cup dried cranberries
- 1/4 cup diced red onion
- 1/4 cup diced celery
- 2 tablespoons honey Dijon mustard
- 1 tablespoon olive oil mayonnaise
- 1/2 teaspoon salt
- 1/4 teaspoon freshly ground black pepper

In a medium bowl, combine the chicken, apples, cranberries, onion, and celery and mix well.

In a small bowl, combine the mustard, mayonnaise, salt, and pepper and whisk together until well blended.

Stir the dressing into the chicken mixture until thoroughly combined.

Serves 2.

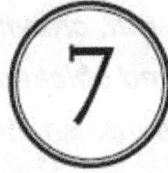

SNACKS

Nutty Apple Salad

This light and crunchy salad is full of fruit and nuts, and appeals to both kids and adults. It keeps well for up to two days, and because it doesn't get soggy, it's perfect to pack in a lunch box.

- 6 firm apples, such as Gala or Golden Delicious, peeled, cored, and sliced
- 1 tablespoon freshly squeezed lemon juice
- 2 kiwis, peeled and diced
- 1/2 cup sliced strawberries
- 1/2 cup packaged shredded coleslaw mix, without dressing
- 1/2 cup walnut halves

- 1/4 cup slivered almonds
- 1/4 cup balsamic vinegar
- 1/4 cup extra-virgin olive oil
- 2 tablespoons sesame seeds, plus more for garnish (optional)
- 1/4 teaspoon salt
- 1/4 teaspoon freshly ground black pepper

In a medium bowl, toss the apple slices with the lemon juice to prevent browning. Add the kiwis, strawberries, coleslaw mix, walnuts, and almonds and toss well to mix.

In a small bowl, whisk together the balsamic vinegar, olive oil, and sesame seeds and season with salt and pepper.

Pour the dressing over the salad and toss to coat.

To serve, spoon into small bowls and top with additional sesame seeds if desired.

Serves 4.

Kale Chips

Kale is chock-full of iron, folate, potassium, and vitamin C, and when crisped in the oven makes a delicate and delicious snack that puts potato chips to shame. These don't keep very well, but they won't need to.

- 2 large bunches kale, ribs removed
- 1 tablespoon extra-virgin olive oil
- 1 teaspoon salt

Arrange the oven racks in the upper and middle positions. Preheat the oven to 250°F. Line 2 baking sheets with aluminum foil.

Rinse the kale and dry very well with a towel or salad spinner. Tear into large pieces.

Toss the kale with the olive oil and arrange in a single layer on the baking sheets. Sprinkle with salt.

Bake for 20 minutes and then use tongs to gently turn each leaf over. Bake until dry and crisp, another 10 to 15 minutes. Serve warm.

Serves 2 to 4.

Sweet Potato Fries

Sweet potatoes have far more vitamin A and C and far less starch than white potatoes and make for wonderfully flavorful oven fries. Experiment with different seasonings, such as mild curry, cayenne, or garlic powder, to find your favorite combination. Instead of ketchup, dip these in a little olive oil flavored with black pepper.

- 4 large sweet potatoes, peeled and cut into finger-like strips
- 2 tablespoons extra-virgin olive oil
- 1/2 teaspoon salt
- 1/2 teaspoon freshly ground black pepper

Preheat the oven to 350°F. Line a baking sheet with aluminum foil. Toss the potatoes in a large bowl with the olive oil, salt, and pepper.

Arrange the potatoes in a single layer on the baking sheet and bake until brown at the edges, about 40 minutes. Serve piping hot.

Serves 4.

Heart-Healthful Trail Mix

This trail mix takes just a few minutes to throw together, keeps for weeks in an airtight container, and is loaded with heart-healthful ingredients. Take it to work or the gym for a quick pick-me-up.

- 1 cup raw almonds
- 1 cup walnut halves
- 1 cup pumpkin seeds
- 1 cup dried apricots, cut into thin strips
- 1 cup dried cherries, roughly chopped
- 1 cup golden raisins
- 2 tablespoons extra-virgin olive oil
- 1 teaspoon salt

Preheat the oven to 300°F. Line a baking sheet with aluminum foil.

In a large bowl, combine the almonds, walnuts, pumpkin seeds, apricots, cherries, and raisins. Pour the olive oil over all and toss well with clean hands. Add salt and toss again to distribute.

Pour the nut mixture onto the baking sheet in a single layer and bake until the fruits begin to brown, about 30 minutes. Cool on the baking sheet to room temperature.

Store in a large airtight container or zipper-top plastic bag.

Serves 10 to 12.

Pesto Cucumber Boats

This appetizer packs a big flavor punch for such a light dish. It's ideal for a cocktail party or dinner buffet. For a slightly different taste and crisper texture, substitute large celery stalks for the cucumber. The pesto is made with walnuts instead of pine nuts for a slight twist; any leftovers can be stored in an airtight container in the refrigerator for up to a week.

- 3 medium cucumbers
- 1/4 teaspoon salt
- 1 packed cup fresh basil leaves
- 1 garlic clove, minced
- 1/4 cup walnut pieces
- 1/4 cup grated Parmesan cheese
- 1/4 cup extra-virgin olive oil
- 1/2 teaspoon paprika

Cut each cucumber in half lengthwise and again in half crosswise to make 4 stocky pieces. Use a spoon to remove the seeds and hollow out a shallow trough in each piece. Lightly salt each piece and set aside on a platter.

In a blender or food processor, combine the basil, garlic, walnuts, Parmesan cheese, and olive oil and blend until smooth.

Use a spoon to spread pesto into each cucumber "boat" and sprinkle each with paprika. Serve.

Serves 4 to 6.

Citrus-Kissed Melon

Here's a fruit salad that is as refreshing as a dip in the ocean. It will keep in the fridge for up to three days, so it's an ideal make-ahead snack. For variety, experiment with different types of melon every time you make this treat.

- 2 cups cubed melon, such as Crenshaw, Sharlyn, or honeydew
- 2 cups cubed cantaloupe
- 1/2 cup freshly squeezed orange juice
- 1/4 cup freshly squeezed lime juice
- 1 tablespoon orange zest

In a large bowl, combine the melon cubes. In a small bowl, whisk together the orange juice, lime juice, and orange zest and pour over the fruit.

Cover and refrigerate for at least 4 hours, stirring occasionally. Serve chilled.

Serves 4.

Spicy-Sweet Roasted Walnuts

These tasty walnuts take just a few minutes to prepare and have a spicy kick. Feel free to double the recipe, as these will keep for up to two weeks in an airtight container.

- 4 cups walnut halves
- 2 tablespoons extra-virgin olive oil
- 1 tablespoon mild curry powder
- 1 teaspoon salt
- 1/4 cup lightly packed light brown sugar

Preheat the oven to 250°F. Line a baking sheet with aluminum foil.

In a large bowl, use clean hands to toss the walnuts with the olive oil to coat. Sprinkle with curry powder and salt and toss again.

Spread out the walnuts on the baking sheet and bake for 15 minutes. Remove from the oven and allow to cool just until warm to the touch, about 10 minutes.

Sprinkle the warm walnuts with the brown sugar and allow to cool to room temperature before storing in an airtight container.

Serves 8 to 10.

Café Cooler

Try this refreshing coffee drink as a pick-me-up in the middle of the day or on a summer evening. It's best made with espresso, but you can substitute strong coffee if you prefer.

- Ice cubes
- 2 cups low-fat milk
- 1/2 teaspoon ground cinnamon
- 1/2 teaspoon pure vanilla extract
- 1 cup espresso, cooled to room temperature
- 4 teaspoons sugar (optional)

Fill four tall glasses with ice cubes.

In a blender, combine the milk, cinnamon, and vanilla and blend until frothy.

Pour the milk over the ice cubes and top each drink with one-quarter of the espresso. If using sugar, stir it into the espresso until it has dissolved. Serve immediately, with chilled teaspoons for stirring.

Serves 4.

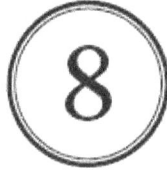

Dilly Baked Salmon

Salmon paired with dill is a culinary classic, and it's especially delicious prepared with a touch of citrus and a little olive oil. Baking fish in foil packets maximizes flavor and minimizes mess.

- 4 (6-ounce) salmon filets
- 2 tablespoons extra-virgin olive oil
- 1/2 teaspoon salt

- Juice of large Valencia orange or tangerine
- 4 teaspoons orange or tangerine

- 1/4 teaspoon freshly ground black zest pepper
- 4 tablespoons chopped fresh dill

Preheat the oven to 375°F. Prepare four 10-inch-long pieces of aluminum foil.

Rub each salmon filet on both sides with the olive oil. Season each with salt and pepper and place one in the center of each piece of foil.

Drizzle the orange juice over each piece of fish and top with 1 teaspoon orange zest and 1 tablespoon dill.

For each packet, fold the two long sides of the foil together and then fold the short ends in to make a packet. Make sure to leave about 2 inches of air space within the foil so the fish can steam. Place the packets on a baking sheet.

Bake for 15 minutes. Open the packets carefully (they will be very steamy), transfer the fish to 4 serving plates, and pour the sauce over the top of each.

Serves 4.

Herb-Roasted Whole Chicken

For a weekend family dinner or a small dinner party, nothing beats the aroma and appeal of a crispy, golden roasted chicken. If there are only one or two of you at home, have this for dinner one night and enjoy the leftovers in salads, sandwiches, or pasta dishes.

- 1 (3to 31/2-pound) roasting chicken
- 1 tablespoon extra-virgin olive oil
- 4 rosemary sprigs
- 6 thyme sprigs
- 4 fresh sage leaves
- 1 bay leaf
- 1 teaspoon freshly squeezed lemon juice
- 1 teaspoon salt
- 1/2 teaspoon freshly ground black pepper

Preheat the oven to 400°F. Place a rack inside a large roasting pan.

Rub the olive oil all over the chicken. As you do, gently loosen the skin over the breast to form a pocket.

Slide half of the rosemary and thyme sprigs underneath the skin over the breast, and put the sage leaves, bay leaf, and remaining sprigs inside the cavity.

Rub with the lemon juice and season with salt and pepper.

Roast until an instant-read thermometer inserted into the thigh registers 165°F, 50 to 60 minutes. Remove from the oven and allow to rest for 10 minutes before carving.

Serves 6.

Penne with Roasted Vegetables

Penne has enough heft to hold its own when combined with chunky ingredients. Paired with caramelized roasted veggies, it makes a filling, nutritious meal.

- 1 large butternut squash, peeled and diced
- 1 large zucchini, diced
- 1 large yellow onion, chopped
- 2 tablespoons extra-virgin olive oil
- 1/2 teaspoon salt
- 1/2 teaspoon freshly ground black pepper

- 1 teaspoon paprika
- 1/2 teaspoon garlic powder
- 1 pound whole-grain penne
- 1/2 cup dry white wine or chicken stock
- 2 tablespoons grated Parmesan cheese

Preheat the oven to 400°F. Line a baking sheet with aluminum foil.

In a large bowl, toss the vegetables with the olive oil, then spread them out on the baking sheet. Sprinkle the vegetables with the salt, pepper, paprika, and garlic powder and bake just until fork-tender, 25 to 30 minutes.

Meanwhile, bring a large stockpot of water to a boil over high heat and cook the penne according to the package instructions until al dente (still slightly firm). Drain but do not rinse.

Place 1/2 cup of the roasted vegetables and the wine or stock in a blender or food processor and blend until smooth.

Place the purée in a large skillet and heat over medium-high heat. Add the pasta and cook, stirring, just until heated through.

Serve the pasta and sauce topped with the roasted vegetables. Sprinkle with Parmesan cheese.

Serves 6.

Fettuccine with Tomatoes and Pesto

Bursting with ripe tomatoes and fresh basil, this dish is the very essence of summer. Keep the heavier tomato sauces for winter, and make this your warm-weather go-to dinner. If you make the pesto in advance, it's a quick and delicious way to have a relaxing dinner after a busy day.

- 1 pound whole-grain fettuccine
- 4 Roma tomatoes, diced
- 2 teaspoons tomato paste
- 1 cup vegetable broth
- 2 garlic cloves, minced
- 1 tablespoon chopped fresh oregano
- 1/2 teaspoon salt
- 1 packed cup fresh basil leaves
- 1/4 cup extra-virgin olive oil
- 1/4 cup grated Parmesan cheese
- 1/4 cup pine nuts

Bring a large stockpot of water to a boil over high heat, and cook the fettuccine according to the package instructions until al dente (still slightly firm). Drain but do not rinse.

Meanwhile, in a large, heavy skillet, combine the tomatoes, tomato paste, broth, garlic, oregano, and salt and stir well. Cook over medium heat for 10 minutes.

In a blender or food processor, combine the basil, olive oil, Parmesan cheese, and pine nuts and blend until smooth.

Stir the pesto into the tomato mixture. Add the pasta and cook, stirring frequently, just until the pasta is well coated and heated through.

Serve immediately.

Serves 4.

Hearty Chicken and Vegetable Soup

You'll think this soup simmered all day, but it takes only thirty minutes to prepare. Refrigerate leftovers in the fridge for up to three days or in the freezer for up to a month so you'll always have some on hand for a quick meal.

- 1 teaspoon extra-virgin olive oil
- 1 medium yellow onion, diced
- 1 large carrot, peeled and diced
- 1 celery stalk, peeled and diced
- 2 (6-ounce) boneless, skinless chicken breasts, cut into 1-inch pieces
- 1 medium zucchini, diced
- 2 yellow squash, diced
- 1/2 cup chopped fresh parsley, plus extra for garnish
- 1 teaspoon chopped fresh oregano
- 1 teaspoon chopped fresh basil
- 1/2 teaspoon salt
- 1/4 teaspoon freshly ground black pepper
- 2 cups chicken stock

In a large, heavy skillet, heat the olive oil over medium-high heat. Add the onion, carrot, and celery and sauté, stirring frequently, for 5 minutes. Add the chicken and continue to sauté for another 10 minutes, stirring often.

Add the zucchini and squash, then the parsley, oregano, basil, salt, and pepper. Sauté for 5 minutes, reduce the heat to medium, and pour in the stock. Cover and cook for an additional 10 minutes.

To serve, ladle into bowls and garnish with additional parsley.

Serves 2.

Flank Steak Spinach Salad

Flank steak is an especially lean cut, which makes it a top choice for those occasional meals when you'd like to serve red meat. Incorporating it into a salad makes the meat, and your grocery dollar, go a lot farther.

- 1 pound flank steak
- 1 teaspoon extra-virgin olive oil
- 1 tablespoon garlic powder
- 1/2 teaspoon salt
- 1/2 teaspoon freshly ground black pepper

- 4 cups baby spinach leaves
- 10 cherry tomatoes, halved
- 10 cremini or white mushrooms, sliced
- 1 small red onion, thinly sliced
- 1/2 red bell pepper, thinly sliced

Preheat the broiler. Line a baking sheet with aluminum foil.

Rub the top of the flank steak with the olive oil, garlic powder, salt, and pepper and let sit for 10 minutes before placing under the broiler. Broil for 5 minutes on each side for medium rare. Allow the meat to rest on a cutting board for 10 minutes.

Meanwhile, in a large bowl, combine the spinach, tomatoes, mushrooms, onion, and bell pepper and toss well.

To serve, divide the salad among 4 dinner plates. Slice the steak on the diagonal and place 4 to 5 slices on top of each salad. Serve with your favorite vinaigrette.

Serves 4.

Oven-Poached Cod

Cod is a firm, mild fish that is a terrific source of omega-3 fats. It cooks up easily, takes on the flavors of other ingredients readily, and isn't too expensive, so it's particularly suited to seafood novices. If you have an oven-safe skillet, this is a one-pan meal that makes for easy cleanup.

- 4 (6-ounce) cod filets
- 1/2 teaspoon salt
- 1/2 teaspoon freshly ground black pepper
- 1/2 cup dry white wine
- 1/2 cup seafood or vegetable stock

- 2 garlic cloves, minced
- 1 bay leaf
- 1 teaspoon chopped fresh sage
- 4 rosemary sprigs for garnish

Preheat the oven to 375°F.

Season each filet with salt and pepper and place in a large ovenproof skillet or baking pan. Add the wine, stock, garlic, bay leaf, and sage and cover. Bake until the fish flakes easily with a fork, about 20 minutes.

Use a spatula to remove the filet from the skillet. Place the poaching liquid over high heat and cook, stirring frequently, until reduced by half, about 10 minutes. (Do this in a small saucepan if you used a baking pan.)

To serve, place a filet on each plate and drizzle with the reduced poaching liquid. Garnish each with a fresh rosemary sprig.

Serves 4.

Mussels with White Wine

Mussels simmered in white wine is a traditional dish served all over the Mediterranean. It's ready in minutes, very impressive, and cannot be beat for pure comfort when served with crusty bread for sopping the juices.

- 4 pounds fresh, live mussels
- 2 cups dry white wine
- 1/2 teaspoon sea salt
- 6 garlic cloves, minced
- 4 teaspoons diced shallot
- 1/2 cup chopped fresh parsley, divided
- 4 tablespoons extra-virgin olive oil
- Juice of 1/2 lemon

In a large colander, scrub and rinse the mussels under cold water. Discard any mussels that do not close when tapped. Use a paring knife to remove the beard from each mussel.

In a large stockpot over medium-high heat, bring the wine, salt, garlic, shallots, and 1/4 cup of the parsley to a steady simmer.

Add the mussels, cover, and simmer just until all of the mussels open, 5 to 7 minutes. Do not overcook.

Using a slotted spoon, divide the mussels among 4 large, shallow bowls.

Add the olive oil and lemon juice to the pot, stir, and pour the broth over the mussels. Garnish each serving with 1 tablespoon of the remaining fresh parsley and serve with a crusty, wholegrain baguette.

Serves 4.

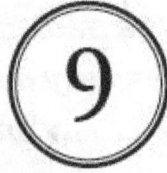

9

DESSERT

Summer Fruit Granita

This refreshing dessert tastes like summer in a bowl. Granita is exceptionally simple to make, and its fresh flavor beats anything you can get at the ice cream shop.

- 1/4 cup sugar
- 1 cup fresh strawberries
- 1 cup fresh raspberries
- 1 cup fresh blackberries
- 1 teaspoon freshly squeezed lemon juice

In a small saucepan, bring 1 cup water to a boil over high heat. Add the sugar and stir well until dissolved.

Remove the pan from the heat, add the berries and lemon juice, and cool to room temperature. Once cooled, place the fruit in a blender or food processor and blend on high until smooth.

Pour the puree into a shallow glass baking dish and place in the freezer for 1 hour. Stir with a fork and freeze for 30 minutes, then repeat.

To serve, use an ice cream scoop to portion the granita into dessert dishes.

Serves 4.

Dark Chocolate Hot Chocolate

Dark chocolate that contains at least 70 percent cacao is what you need for this recipe. It's a surprisingly good source of heart-healthful antioxidants and is sinfully rich. This recipe is inspired by the very thick and creamy hot chocolate served in Italy and France.

- 4 cups low-fat milk
- 2 teaspoons sugar
- 4 (1-ounce) squares dark chocolate
- 1/2 teaspoon salt
- 1/2 teaspoon ground cinnamon
- 1/4 teaspoon chili powder

In a medium, heavy saucepan, heat the milk and sugar over low heat until it reaches a simmer.

Place the dark chocolate, salt, cinnamon, and chili powder in a medium bowl and pour just enough hot milk over the chocolate to cover.

Return the pan to the heat and reduce the heat to low.

Whisk the hot milk and chocolate together until the chocolate has melted, then pour the mixture into the remaining milk in the saucepan, whisking constantly.

To serve, divide among 4 mugs.

Serves 4.

Home-Baked Biscotti

Biscotti are a favorite sweet in Italy, particularly served alongside espresso. Happily, they're one of the easiest treats to bake. These keep well in an airtight container for up to two weeks, so double the recipe to make enough to last a while. These are also wonderful dipped in red wine.

- 2 cups whole-wheat flour
- 3/4 cup sugar
- 1 teaspoon baking powder
- 1/4 teaspoon salt
- 3/4 cup slivered almonds

- 3 large eggs
- 2 tablespoons pure almond extract
- 1 teaspoon pure vanilla extract
- 1 teaspoon extra-virgin olive oil

Place an oven rack in the middle position and preheat the oven to 275°F.

In a large bowl, combine the flour, sugar, baking powder, salt, and almonds and stir with a wooden spoon until well combined.

In a small bowl, whisk together the eggs, almond extract, and vanilla.

Pour the egg mixture into the dry ingredients and use a wooden spoon to mix well, stirring for about 2 minutes to ensure that the ingredients are well combined.

Use your hands to grease a baking sheet with the olive oil and then use your greased hands to spread the dough onto the baking sheet in a rectangle about 11 x 4 inches.

Bake for 45 minutes, remove from the oven, and use a sharp, greased knife to cut the rectangle crosswise into 1/2-inch slices. Lay the slices cut side up about 1/2 inch apart and return the baking sheet to the oven.

Bake until the cut sides are quite dry, about 20 minutes.

Cool on the baking sheet to room temperature, then store in an airtight container.

Makes about 20 biscotti.

Chocolate-Dipped Fruit Bites

Here's a treat that is fun to make and even more fun to eat. It's perfect for when you have little helpers in the kitchen, but you may need to make extra to replace the ones that get eaten along the way! Any leftovers will keep in an airtight container in the refrigerator for up to two days.

- 1/2 cup semisweet chocolate chips
- 1/4 cup low-fat milk
- 1/2 teaspoon pure vanilla extract
- 1/2 teaspoon ground nutmeg
- 1/4 teaspoon salt
- 2 kiwis, peeled and sliced
- 1 cup honeydew melon chunks (about 2-inch chunks)
- 1 pound whole strawberries

Place the chocolate chips in a small bowl.

In another small bowl, microwave the milk until hot, about 30 seconds. Pour the milk over the chocolate chips and let sit for 1 minute, then whisk until the chocolate is melted and smooth. Stir in the vanilla, nutmeg, and salt and allow to cool for 5 minutes.

Line a baking sheet with wax paper. Dip each piece of fruit halfway into the chocolate, tap gently to remove excess chocolate, and place the fruit on the baking sheet.

Once all the fruit has been dipped, allow it to sit until dry, about 30 minutes. Arrange on a platter and serve.

Serves 4 to 6.

Baked Pears in Red Wine Sauce

Prepare this elegant dessert when you're celebrating a special occasion or want to impress some dinner guests. It looks and tastes fancy but is it's not simple to make. If you like, bake the pears a few hours ahead of time and let them sit at room temperature. Just reheat the sauce before serving.

- 4 just-ripe firm pears, such as Bosc or Anjou
- 1 cup sweet red wine, such as port or Beaujolais Nouveau
- 1 cinnamon stick
- 2 teaspoons light brown sugar
- 1/2 teaspoon pure almond extract
- 4 mint sprigs for garnish

Preheat the oven to 325°F.

Peel the pears, leaving the core and stem intact. Cut a slice from the bottom of each to allow them to stand easily. Place the pears in a small baking dish.

In a small saucepan, combine the red wine, cinnamon stick, and brown sugar and heat over low heat just until it reaches a simmer. Stir in the almond extract, remove the cinnamon stick, and pour the liquid into the baking dish. Slide the dish into the oven, being careful not to tip the pears.

Bake until the pears are golden and fork-tender, about 1 hour. The bottom one-third to onehalf will be a deep red.

Gently transfer the pears to a platter and pour the red wine mixture back into the saucepan. Heat over medium heat and simmer until reduced by half, about 15 minutes. Remove the pan from the heat and allow the sauce to cool for 10 minutes.

To serve, place each pear in a shallow dessert bowl and pour a little red wine sauce around it. Garnish with fresh mint.

Serves 4.

Roasted Honey-Cinnamon Apples

For this dish you'll want to look for Stayman Winesap or Gala apples, which are firm enough to hold up to roasting and maintain their slightly tart flavor. This is a simple but delicious way to make the most of this healthful fall fruit.

- 1 teaspoon extra-virgin olive oil
- 4 firm apples, peeled, cored, and sliced
- 1/2 teaspoon salt
- 11/2 teaspoons ground cinnamon, divided
- 2 tablespoons low-fat milk
- 2 tablespoons honey

Preheat the oven to 375°F. Grease a small casserole dish with the olive oil.

In a medium bowl, toss the apple slices with the salt and 1/2 teaspoon of the cinnamon. Spread the apples in the baking dish and bake for 20 minutes.

Meanwhile, in a small saucepan, heat the milk, honey, and remaining 1 teaspoon cinnamon over medium heat, stirring frequently. When it reaches a simmer, remove the pan from the heat and cover to keep warm.

Divide the apple slices between 2 dessert plates and pour the sauce over the apples. Serve warm.

Serves 2.

Grilled Pineapple and Melon

Grilling fruit caramelizes its natural sugars and really brings out the fruit's flavor. It's the ideal dessert for an afternoon cookout, but you can just as easily prepare this on an indoor grill.

- 8 fresh pineapple rings, rind removed
- 8 watermelon triangles, with rind
- 1 tablespoon honey
- 1/2 teaspoon freshly ground black pepper

Preheat an outdoor grill or a grill pan over high heat.

Drizzle the fruit slices with honey and sprinkle one side of each piece with pepper. Grill for 5 minutes, turn, and grill for another 2 minutes. Serve.

Serves 4.

Red Grapefruit Granita

Red grapefruit is a tasty source of vitamin C and a host of other important antioxidants, including resveratrol. It makes a most refreshing granita, the perfect ending to an outdoor dinner on a warm summer evening.

- 3 cups red grapefruit sections
- 1 cup freshly squeezed red grapefruit juice
- 1/4 cup honey
- 1 tablespoon freshly squeezed lime juice
- Fresh basil leaves for garnish

Remove as much pith (white part) and membrane as possible from the grapefruit segments.

Combine all ingredients except the basil in a blender or food processor and pulse just until smooth.

Pour the mixture into a shallow glass baking dish and place in the freezer for 1 hour. Stir with a fork and freeze for another 30 minutes, then repeat.

To serve, scoop into small dessert glasses and garnish with fresh basil leaves.

Serves 4 to 6.

CONCLUSION

The Mediterranean diet isn't just a way to eat, it's a way to love eating. Commit to not only following the diet, but following the example of a culture where fresh, seasonal ingredients are respected and prized, where meals are simply prepared and generously shared, and where time is spent lingering over food, wine, and conversation.

Eating the Mediterranean way can not only improve your health and help you lose weight, it can also encourage you to slow down, at least two or three times a day, and take a break from a hectic schedule and a busy life.

Have fun exploring the Mediterranean diet; enjoy spending weekends at your local farmers' market and make an adventure out of trying new ingredients. Build more social time into your week by sharing these simple but delicious dishes with your family and friends.

The Mediterranean diet isn't just about healthful living; it's about joyful living!

REFERENCES

Domínguez, L.J., M. Bes-Rastrollo, C. de la Fuente-Arrillaga, et al. "Similar prediction of decreased total mortality, diabetes incidence or cardiovascular events using relativeand absolute-component Mediterranean diet score: The SUN cohort." *Nutrition, Metabolism and Cardiovascular Diseases* , March 6, 2012.

Estruch R., E. Ros, J. Salas-Salvadó, et al. "Primary prevention of cardiovascular disease with a Mediterranean diet." *The New England Journal of Medicine* , February 25, 2013.

Fernández-Real, J.M., M. Bulló, J.M. Moreno-Navarrete, et al. "A Mediterranean diet enriched with olive oil is associated with higher serum total osteocalcin levels in elderly men at high cardiovascular risk." *Journal of Clinical Endocrinology and Metabolism* , October 2012: 3792–98.

Gardener H., C.B. Wright, Y. Gu, et al. "Mediterranean-style diet and risk of ischemic stroke, myocardial infarction, and vascular death: the Northern Manhattan Study." *The American Journal of Clinical Nutrition* , vol. 94 no. 6 (December 2011): 1458–64.

Gil, A., R.M. Ortega, J. Maldonado. "Wholegrain cereals and bread: a duet of the Mediterranean diet for the prevention of chronic diseases." *Public Health Nutrition* , 2011: 2316–22.

Haber, B. "The Mediterranean Diet: a view from history." *The American Journal of Clinical Nutrition* , vol. 66 no. 4 (October 1997): 10535–75.

Harvard School of Public Health. "Close adherence to a traditional Mediterranean diet promotes longevity." Press release, June 25, 2003.

http://archive.sph.harvard.edu/press-releases/archives/2003-releases/press06252003.html (accessed March 20, 2013) .

Kromhout, D., A. Menotti, B. Bloemberg, et al. "Dietary saturated and trans fatty acids and cholesterol and 25-year mortality from coronary heart disease: the Seven Countries Study." *Preventive Medicine* , vol. 24 no. 3 (May 1995): 308–15.

Nordmann, A.J., K. Suter-Zimmermann, H.C. Bucher, et al. "Meta-analysis comparing Mediterranean to low-fat diets for modification of cardiovascular risk factors." *The American Journal of Medicine* , vol. 124 no. 9 (September 2011): 841–51.

Scarmeas, N., J. Luchsinger, R. Mayeaux, et al. "Mediterranean diet and Alzheimer disease mortality." *Neurology* , vol. 69 no. 11 (September 2007): 1084–93.

UNESCO.org. "Mediterranean diet," 2010. http://www.unesco.org/culture/ich/en/RL/00394 (accessed March 20, 2012).

U.S. National Library of Medicine, National Institutes of Health. "Wine and heart health." MedLine Plus web site, 2012. http://www.nlm.nih.gov/medlineplus/ency/article/001963.htm (accessed March 20, 2013).

Willet, W.C., F. Sacks, A. Trichopoulou, et al. "Mediterranean diet pyramid: a cultural model for healthy eating." *American Journal of Clinical Nutrition* , vol. 61 no. 6 (June 1995): 14025–65 .

www.ingramcontent.com/pod-product-compliance
Lightning Source LLC
Chambersburg PA
CBHW080628030426
42336CB00018B/3123